PLANT BASED

FOR BEGINNERS

A Step by Step Guide for Weight

Loss with A Natural Meal Plan

DELIA FLOWERDAY

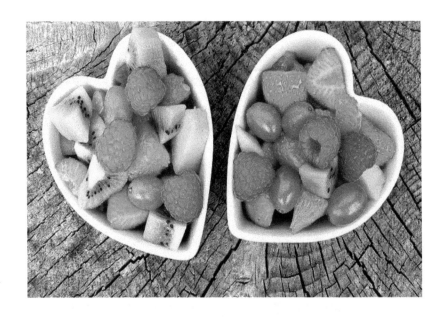

Table of Contents

1. Introduction

Some of the most popular vegan diets that people have either been wanting to try or have been curious about are the 'raw till four diet' which has been made amazingly popular due to a vegan on a viral video site. As of now, I believe there is a following of about eight thousand or more, plant-based vegan. Most of the people that use this diet have said that they've tried others, and this was the best for them; low carb vegan such as keto or paleo; and the engine two diets on the opposite side of keto. Some prefer high carb low-fat diets, the detox vegan diet, or even the junk food vegan diet which they love because it proves that being a vegan you don't have to just stick to healthy 'boring' food but instead you can eat amazingly tasty food as well.

One of the most obvious benefits of vegans is that they tend to be skinnier and able to better maintain a healthier weight than most meat eaters. As with any diet, this depends on what you eat. There are many meat and cheese substitutes that are vegan, but some can be high in calories and other things that can make you gain weight if that's all you're eating or junk food related items. Many companies are understanding that more people are becoming vegan and therefore want to put out substitutes and many people fill up on these because they don't do the proper research as to how they should be eating. This causes weight gain. Another problem for new vegans is they listen to fad diet people. An example of this is viral video sites. A lot of the information from these videos is solid and well informed; others, not so much.

There have been people on these channels telling people to eat over five thousand calories a day in fruit and only to exercise an hour. Obviously, this may not be the best advice because that's far too much sugar and calories with only one hour of exercise. You wouldn't be able to burn off that many calories with so little workout time. This could make you balloon up and have a host of health issues. Another fad diet that has come under scrutiny is the 'raw till four' simply because nutritionists have said it's dangerous especially if you're following some of the people on these viral video sites especially when they take it to some of the far extremes. So it's important to know what it is you're doing with your diet. Eating properly can make a vegan skinnier; eating improperly will not.

Since you will no longer be eating meat or dairy, you are likely to be eating foods with a lot less saturated fat. Saturated fat is linked to high cholesterol and increased risk of heart disease. Lower blood pressure is another great benefit of cutting animal products out of your life.

2. What is a plant-based diet?

The question is more like this: what is the difference between a plant-based diet and veganism?

Both food approaches do not involve meat consumption. But if vegans are ethically motivated, those who follow a plant-based diet also reject everything that is processed on an industrial and unhealthy level.

Vegans refrain from eating any animal product. According to the vegan society: "veganism is a way of life that tries to exclude, as far as possible and practicable, all forms of exploitation and cruelty to animals for food, clothing or any other purpose" (the vegan society, n.d).

This means that many vegans do not even buy leather goods and their diet is mostly an ethical philosophy, which excludes the exploitation of animals in all aspects of life. However, it does not mean that they necessarily eat unprocessed foods. The vegan person does not reject any industrially processed products, such as snacks (like oreos), ice cream, or fizzy drinks that are vegan-friendly.

However, a plant-based diet is based on the consumption of fruit, vegetables, and whole grains and avoiding (or minimizing) the intake of animal products and processed foods. This means that even vegan desserts made with refined sugar or bleached flour are not included in a plant-based diet. In short, both diets avoid eating hamburgers (the kind with meat or chicken patties), but for different reasons: vegans because they do not eat meat and those who follow a plant-based diet because they do not eat processed foods and hydrogenated fats, and do so for health reasons.

3. The science of plant based diet eating healthy

While there is no doubt that humans were meant to be eating fruits, vegetables and nuts from the beginning, a shift took place that introduced a large confusion, mixing humans with the omnivore species. Scientifically speaking, a plant-based diet is much more beneficial and less harmful for humans, which is why it is recommended to shift from meat to whole grains, legumes, vegetables and other nutritional foods of this kind.

Switching to a plant based diet is beneficial for many reasons. If you are suffering from any kind of illnesses or have obesity issues, you should focus on a plant based diet as a way to better your health and reduce your symptoms, if not cure the illness completely. Nutrition is a powerful tool that can be used for great purposes, such as helping relieve pain and health problems, improving metabolism and the immune system, as well as strengthen your body and improve your mood.

Even if you do not have any health-related problems, you should transition to a plant based diet as a means of preventive health building. The natural ingredients such as fruits, legumes or vegetables are full of nutritional values needed for the everyday functioning of our systems. In all cases, whole food is always better than processed food, as it does not contain any chemicals or unnatural substances that could be harmful to our health.

Besides boosting your health, a plant-based diet can decrease the risks of many diseases, among them the most serious ones such as heart diseases, type 2 diabetes and certain types of cancers. Many studies at research facilities have proven these statements to be correct, such as, for example, a study conducted in JAMA Internal Medicine, which tracked over 70 000 people and their eating habits. This study has proven that a plant-based diet can significantly improve your health and lengthen your life as well. Therefore, switching to a plant based diet is one of the best things you can do for yourself and your overall well-being.

People who consume plant-based products have a lower risk of developing diseases or having strokes because of the fiber, vitamins and minerals that come along with a plant-based diet. The fiber, vitamins and minerals, as well as healthy fats, are essential substances your body needs in order to function properly. A plant-based diet thus improves the blood lipid levels and better your brain health as well. There is a significant decrease in bad cholesterol in people who follow a plant-based diet.

It is never too late to change your diet! Whether you are 18, 36 or 50, it is still recommended to switch to a plant-based diet, as it is never too late to do so! These diets have quick and effective results that you will be noticing even after the first week of eating only plant-based meals. The first results you will notice will be the sense of accomplishment and satisfaction that comes with following a healthy diet. You will notice your mood has improved, in addition to not feeling heavy after a meal, but instead feeling full and satisfied and yet energetic. After a period of following a plant-based diet, you will begin to notice the health benefits of doing so. Your health-related problems will be reduced and you will feel a significant relief in terms of pains or discomfort you have been having.

What is important to know when switching to a plant-based diet is that you are not going to be on any kind of deprivation diet. Many people relate a plant-based diet as a diet where you are depriving yourself of meat and dairy. However, when you switch to a plant-based diet you will not feel like you are missing anything, since your taste will adapt to your new eating habits. This will lead to you finding foods delicious that you may have even disliked before. The human body is adapting constantly to the different inputs, and after a while, plant-based food will feel tasty and natural to you. The foods prepared of the healthy, nutritional ingredients are very delicious, especially if you follow the right recipes. Stick through this diet guide to learn some great plant based diet recipes you can include in your transition program. Once you see the benefits of the plant based diet and try some of the specialties, you will never want to go back to your old eating habits again.

Transitioning from a meat to a plant based diet is not as difficult as everyone thinks. You can do it gradually, by increasing your fruit and vegetable intake while decreasing your meat and dairy intake. Minimizing meat consumption at first will make the transition seem effortless later, as you don't have to introduce drastic changes immediately. Instead of meat and dairy, you should start consuming the following foods:

fruits such as apples, bananas, grapes, etc.

vegetables such as kale, lettuce, peppers, corn, etc.

tubers such as potatoes, beets, carrots, etc.

whole grains such as rice, oats, millet, whole wheat, etc.

legumes such as kidney beans, black beans, chickpeas, etc.

Therefore, your diet will be based on fruits, vegetables, tubers, whole grains and legumes. You can start implementing these changes by replacing meat in your favorite recipes and dishes with mushrooms or beans. Gradually, you will completely lose the habit of consuming meat and switch to a full plant based diet. To help your transition process, you should add more calories of legumes, whole grains and vegetables to your everyday routine, as that will make you feel full and thus reduce your desire to eat meat and dairy.

As soon as you start switching your diet you will notice how positively your body reacts to receiving all the nutrients it needs to function properly. The foods you should be focusing on include beans, that is, all legumes, berries, broccoli, cabbage, collards, nuts and kale.

Before we get into the detailed, 4 week program for switching to a plant based diet, here are a few tips that will help you make the transition easily.

Include fruits and vegetables in every meal of the day. Instead of snacking on chocolate bars, switch to fruit or nutritional bars. Remember, an apple a day keeps the doctor away!

Downsize your meat servings gradually. Put less meat on your plate and more veggies. Make sure that ¾ of the plate consists of plant-based ingredients!

You can slowly transition by introducing two or three meat-free days to your week plan. As time goes by you will get used to this system and you will be able to skip meat more often, until fully switching to the plant based diet.

In addition to the many medical benefits of switching to a plant-based diet, there are also some truly powerful and indisputable cosmetic benefits as well. Many studies have shown that there is a significant and strong link between the consumption of dairy products like milk, butter, or cheese, and undesirable skin conditions like acne, eczema, and early signs of aging. Milk contains many similar properties to the hormone testosterone due to other hormones like progesterone making their way into the milk. It is thought that these hormones stimulate the oil glands of the skin, especially the face. An excess of sebum, or oil, is produced and thus acne occurs. This excess oil clogs your pores and can lead to other troublesome skin blemishes such as blackheads and whiteheads. This continuous cycle of clogged pores, blemishes, and acne takes a lot out of your skin and can cause scarring and stress. This can lead to signs of premature aging and skin loses its elasticity and vitality. Many people who switch to a plant-based diet notice an incredibly rapid improvement in the condition of their skin. People who have suffered from acne and started eating plant-based foods have noticed their skin clear significantly. This is in no way by chance. Cutting out or greatly reducing dairy can really help give your skin a new lease on life. If you are struggling with acne and have tried nearly everything under the sun such as harsh chemicals, expensive facials and skin treatments, or countless different brands claiming to heal your skin problems, something as simple as a plant-based diet may be the answer you've been searching for.

Followers of a plant-based diet have also raved about the excellent anti-aging benefits of the diet. Collagen, something our bodies naturally produce in abundance when we are young, is the key factor of what makes skin supple, resilient, firm, and have elasticity. As we get older, collagen production slows and our skin suffers as a result, becoming prone to sagginess and thinness. While this is a natural and inevitable part of life, collagen loss does not have to be so drastic as we age. A plant-based diet has been proven to boost collagen in your body by providing all of the important nutrients and amino acids that make up collagen and how it is produced. In a sense, subscribing to a plant-based diet is kind of like taking a dip in the fountain of youth! Fruits and vegetables like kale, broccoli, asparagus, spinach, grapefruit, lemons, and oranges are chock-full of vitamin C which is an extremely important component in producing the amino acids that make up collagen. The kind of lean protein found in nuts is important in keeping collagen around, adding to skin cell longevity and resilience. Red vegetables like tomatoes, beets, and red peppers all contain lycopene which is a kind of antioxidant that protects skin from the sun while simultaneously increases collagen production. Foods rich in zinc such as certain seeds and whole grains also promote collagen because the mineral repairs damaged cells and reduces inflammation. So many of the plant-based staples contain incredible amounts of all these collagen-boosting nutrients that you do not even have to go out of your way to seek them out. It is all right there in front of you! Looking and feeling younger has never been so easy. It really does start with the internal to make the external radiant and glowing, outer beauty starts from within.

In short, there are no two ways about it - switching to a plant based diet is good for your heart, your health, your mind, and even your physical appearance! The facts of the matter are undeniable. Plant foods contain so many of the incredibly good nutrients that our bodies need to function properly. Making these foods a priority and centering your meals around them rather than just eating vegetables as an occasional side dish or a piece of fruit every now and then makes a huge difference in your health. By eating a diet heavy on meat, dairy, and other animal products and processed foods, it is easy to miss out on the wonderfully beneficial vitamins, minerals, antioxidants, and other nutrients that are in fruits, vegetables, legumes, tubers, grains, nuts, and seeds. Switching to a plant-based diet gives you the opportunity to obtain all of these healthful ingredients that will without a doubt lead you to a better, more fulfilling life.

4. Benefits of a plant based diet

It is essential to understand that a plant-based meal plan does not necessarily mean permanently eliminating animal products from your diet. It involves incorporating more and more plants and vegetables in your diet. It is a way of eating to satisfaction while not denying your body the essential nutrients it requires. Perception is in the mind. Therefore, before one decides to stick to a plant-based meal, it is imperative to feed in your thinking that it is the best for your body, mind, and soul. That way, you'll start developing a taste and liking for the plant-based meal, and with time, you will find it sweet and very fulfilling.

A plant-based meal has been used over the years both for therapeutic or just nutritional value. There are some vegetables which you may not find tasty, delicious, or sweet. If a plant is bitter you can add fresh herb seasoning, and some can even be blended when making a smoothie. Always try to make it in a way that you can comfortably consume because sometimes it's not very sweet to the mouth but very good to the body.

If we eat a lot of plants, it means we are getting vitamins, fiber, and phytochemicals. These are nutrients that our bodies fall short of, thus keeping us away from taking a lot of supplements. While vegan meals emphasize strictly on eating plant-based foods and zero animal products, plant-based meals incorporate animal protein but in minimal quantity. Plant-based meals thus are very accommodative and less restricting thus create a smooth and easy transitioning when one decides to start.

Key principles of a plant-based diet

• a lot of emphasis on whole foods and minimal focus on processed food. Whole foods are mainly plant-based while processed food mostly comprises of animal products. A plant-based diet is high in nutrients and contains fewer calories. For this reason, even when taken in large quantities, it's not easy for someone to gain weight compared to processed foods. The ease in absorption and digestion and the extra fiber helps prevent constipation.

• focuses mostly on the plant, which includes but not limited to fruits, whole grains, vegetables, legumes, nuts, seeds, and vegetables. These should comprise the majority of the food one eats, and one should be very strict to follow the diet. All servings should contain more plants and less animal protein to enjoy the full benefits.

- quality is more important than quantity; by this, i mean fresh, locally available, or organic is healthier and nutritious. You can liaise with local farmers and get fresh farm produce and prepare them at home. Fresh from the farm is more nutritious and very tasty. Green vegetables lose their nutrients with time if not appropriately stored; thus they should be cooked while still green.
- always consume fats that are healthy, avoid refined fats and oil processed with lots of chemicals. Go for unsaturated fats, which are very good and healthy for your heart. Unhealthy fats are hard to absorb and sometimes bring some health risks like blocked arteries and diabetes.
- start your plant-based with breakfast because this is the meal no one would think should have any vegetables at all. You can take fruit salad; add spinach or kale to your eggs or make a cauliflower smoothie. A healthy breakfast every morning is crucial and should be taken with seriousness, especially if one has started a vegetarian diet. It will give your body the energy needed to start and go through the day, thus making your brain active throughout the day.

- experiment with at least one plant every week. It will increase the variety of vegetables you're used to every week. Additionally, it will also boost your nutrients every week but also make you have a variety to choose from, thus reducing restrictions. It will also expose you to a big world of the various plant-based meals and categorize them as in, easy to prepare, favorite, most nutritious, and tastier.

Health benefits of a plant-based meal

Reduce risk of obesity

Across the globe, millions of people are struggling with obesity or weight-related issues. Sometimes it may be due to eating habits, lifestyle, or genetics. Today, people have not succeeded in losing weight. Striving for a realistic exercise routine is crucial as compared to diet pills, which are very harmful to the body.

Clinical research has shown that a more plant-based diet can help decrease obesity, promoting healthy weight loss. A vegan and vegetarian lifestyle has a significantly low risk of obesity or overweight. A plant-based diet often has high fiber, which is good for digestion and prevents constipation. This helps clear the digestive tract, thus raising the body's metabolism. A plant-based diet is a very healthy way to lose weight without worrying so much about your body, not getting the necessary nutrients. It is also important to note; not all vegetarian diets are healthy.

Obesity can cause many health-related complications and in severe cases, can even promote morbidity. So whether you want to lose weight for health reasons or to keep fit then plant-based meals are the best option. If you compare the room food needs in your stomach, you'll realize plant-based meals are take less space. Thus you'll consume fewer calories.

Reduce cancer risk

Cancer cannot be cured by eating a plant-based diet. It will help reduce one's chances of acquiring cancer, but it must go along with healthy habits and behaviors. Some of these healthy behaviors include alcohol limit, exercise, maintaining a body weight that is normal according to one's body mass index (BMI).

A plant-based diet can help prevent a significant percentage of cancer cases and if it can at least prevent then it is a dietary habit worth emulating. The plant-based meal diet should have lots of fruits, beans, nuts, seeds, and grains with some limited animal food that can prevent cancer. Those kinds of diets contain fiber, minerals, and vitamins that hinder the growth of cancerous cells.

Foods to avoid include but not limited to: fast foods like cheeseburgers, sausages, french fries, chicken nuggets, and hot dogs; refined sugar, canned foods, added sugar, artificial sweetener, and processed animal foods. The phytochemicals available in plant-based meals can fight and thwart cancer cells. It is, therefore, essential to replace unhealthy foods with plant-based meals to lead a healthy and more fulfilling life.

Cancer is now a global problem affecting both children and adults, impoverished and wealthy alike, and the cost of treating cancer can drain a family's financial resources. Sometimes, crowdfunding needs to be done to raise the required money for treatment. It is thus essential to adopt the habit of eating a plant-based diet and form it to be part of you until your system gets used to it.

Start with the plants you are familiar with and are locally available in your area. Then as you make it, routinely try new healthy plant-based recipes, and if you work during lunch, consider packing your lunch from home. Processed and unhealthy food in the diet may rapidly increase the growth of cancer cells for cancer patients. Plant-based meals can also be used as a detox, especially when blended. This applies to fruits and vegetables that can be eaten raw.

Low risk of heart disease

Most plant-based meals are heart-healthy in that they favor the general functioning of the heart. Plant-based meals reduce the risk of developing heart-related diseases like high or low blood pressure, heart attack, and liver problems. We need to note, however, that the quality of the foods consumed and the types matter a lot. This is because high-quality nutrients have the necessary nutrients needed for organ functioning, thus making it practical and healthy.

The heart is the central circulatory system, it is responsible for adding oxygen in the blood, then pumping it throughout the body, and when it stops, then one dies. Not all but various heart diseases are associated with unhealthy eating habits, overconsumption of processed food, and lack of exercise. This diet involves eating food with fewer fats. The advantage of this is that it promotes a healthy heart, which can, in turn, lead to a healthy lifestyle. So most cardiovascular diseases can be prevented by adopting a plant-based meal diet.

Low risk of type 2 diabetes

A plant-based diet does not only reduce the risk of getting type two diabetes, but it can also be a very effective way of managing diabetes. Studies have shown that there is a high prevalence of type two diabetes concerning eating patterns consisting of mainly processed food, animal protein, and refined sugars.

A plant-based diet has potential benefits since it improves the resistance of insulin in the body, promoting recommended and healthy body weight. Increased fiber improves food interactions while decreasing the amount of saturated fat in the body. Those who love eating meat are twice as likely at risk of having diabetes later in life as compared to those who eat more plants. Plant-based meals contain significant insulin sensitivity that is high, which is crucial in maintaining the recommended sugar level that is healthy.

Improved digestion

Digestion of food is essential because it determines absorption. A plant based diet is naturally packed with fiber, which is key to proper and better digestion. Fiber brings additional bulk to one's stool while assisting in regulating, thus smooth elimination of undigested food and stool. When absorption is adequate, the body feels functional and active.

When digestion is proper, there is reduced discomfort associated with problems arising from indigestion, overeating, and eating fatty foods that stay longer in the stomach and take longer to digest and absorb. This will mean the necessary and healthy nutrients are easily absorbed in the bloodstream and the wastes comfortably removed without discomfort or pain. Drinking a lot of water as recommended, also eases digestion.

Boost energy naturally

A plant-based diet is very rich in minerals and vitamins, which give people a lot of energy. The nutrients also act as antioxidants, and the healthy proteins and fats boost brain functioning and make one alert. A plant-based diet is easy to digest and has that extra energy that they release to the body, which enables the body to be more active and boost thinking and improves mood. This is the reason why most professional athletes love and prefer plant-based meals.

Fast foods take longer to digest, slows metabolism, and leaves the body weak and inactive, thus can lead to unnecessary weight gain. Natural energy is more effective than energy derived from energy drinks since it is coming due to satisfaction and not an instant boost. Thus it is essential for everyone, not just athletes, to consume lots of plant proteins so that they can have natural energy to carry out daily tasks.

Healthy hair, skin, & nails

This may sound absurd, but it's true; your hair, skin, and nails' health is based 90% on your diet. What you feed your body and go inside your body will be reflected outside. The vitamins and minerals are good for skin, repairs dead cells as well as givse the skin room to breathe. Meat and dairy products can cause inflammation, which will be visible in the skin. But to achieve the smooth surface, be consistent with your plant-based diet, and be patient because the change will not be realized immediately but after a very long time. Your skin can also appear hydrated and not dry; this is a sign of more plant-based meals in the diet.

Plant-based meals & your health

Those who love meat and fast food often struggle when they start a plant-based diet and can sometimes even find it annoying. Doctors will recommend reducing animal protein intake and maximizing on plants, but how many times have we ignored doctors' recommendations? It's not comfortable with the current fast-paced life, which gives no time to prepare a home-cooked meal.

Also, some people stay places far away from farmers or where access to fresh farm produce is not easy; however, there are some tips you can use so that you don't run out of stock and start indulging. You can buy groceries in bulk worth one week and ensure you store them properly. Poor storage can spoil them, thus making them unsuitable for human consumption.

Compared to fast and processed food, plant-based meals can be slightly expensive, that's why some people may be tempted to grab fast food during lunch, which is cheaper and readily available. It is thus useful to look at long term benefits, potential risks, and your state of health. The cost of medication is or maybe even more expensive than plants and vegetables. This long term benefit makes it worth investing in plant-based meals, which are fresh, nutritious, and healthy.

Kindly keep in mind that people who have some of the diseases discussed above are not vegetarian, and this plant-based diet will not prevent one from getting those diseases, but the diet lowers the risk. Your doctor needs to give you consent if you're on medication or if you have some allergies or just for the doctor to provide you with the approval that it's okay to start a plant-based meal.

Some people are allergic to some grains or nuts; you can get an alternative that is healthy and has the same of better nutritional value. Plants should be included from the first meal of the day, which is breakfast. Include as much as you possibly can, make it appetizing and appealing, if you don't know where to start from do not worry since the next chapters have some simple yet effective recipes that you can use. The recipes contain breakfast, lunch, and supper.

If you are doing a plant-based diet for health reasons, bring your family on board if possible, let them know why you have decided to change your eating habits. Chances are, they will be very appreciative and would give the necessary moral support that you need, you'll also be helping them as they will also consume healthy plant meals, thus live healthier fulfilling lives.

Family and friends can also give recommendations on where to get fresh produce; they can motivate and encourage one another. Eating plant-based meals will help you realize a healthy lifestyle. People who live healthy lives, have more fulfilling, and rewarding lives, therefore, they are happier, and less anxious. They are also active and not conscious of their bodies since they are rarely overweight.

Not all plant-based diets are healthy the same way as not all animal protein is harmful. So as you embark on a plant-based diet, confirm and recheck the quality and nutritional values. The best part about a plant-based diet is the low-calorie rate and it is less fatty. Ensure that you take the recommended calories without overindulging or depriving yourself.

The best news with a plant-based diet is you are not permanently restricted from taking animal protein, but you can choose it in very minimal quantities. This is good news for animal protein lovers and makes the meal plan workable and worth trying. The diet is also progressive in the sense that you can start slowly and not necessarily cut on all animal protein intake at one go.

Health workers are currently encouraging people who are not sick to eat healthy so as to boost their immunity and help their body be able to fight some pathogens without medication. It is also interesting to note that medicines are made using herbs and some plants. Why wait to be sick if a plant-based meal can prevent some sickness?

A plant-based diet, therefore, is an essential diet, and if everyone can get started, then we can have a healthier nation. It is one of the most inclusive vegetarian related diets. Different places have different plants depending on the season so you can take advantage of the season and purchase fresh and locally produced and enjoy the raw nutrients.

Also, one can link with local farmers and ensure that you get quality for your money or instead of purchasing immediately from the farm and prepare the same day, thus preserving the nutrients. A plant-based diet is not easy but realistic and doable as long as you put your mind to it. Redefine yourself today and start consuming a plant-based diet.

5. Vegan Superfoods

To be clear, most superfoods are already vegan, but there are some that are particularly high in nutrient content. The following are the top vegan superfoods available today. These should be incorporated into your diet every chance you get. The following are twelve of the best superfoods that you will find at your local grocery store.

Dark Leafy Greens

Kale, swiss chard, spinach, and collard greens are all classed as dark leafy greens and these superfoods should be incorporated into your daily meal plan. Not only are they a great digestive aid due to their high fiber content, but they're also dense sources of vitamins C and K, zinc, calcium, magnesium, iron and folate. They have a high antioxidant profile that assists the body in removing harmful free radicals which in turn reduces the risk of cancer, heart disease, and stroke.

Berries

Nature's little antioxidants are also the most delicious and delicate fruits we know. Berries host an array of benefits to the body and each one has its own special powers:

Strawberries contain more vitamin C than oranges! They are antioxidant rich and provide us with fiber, potassium, anthocyanins, and folate. Strawberries reduce the risk of cancer, are supportive in the control of diabetes, and are great anti-inflammatories.

Blueberries are one of the most antioxidant-rich foods out there. They contain manganese and vitamins C and K, are supportive of cognitive function and mental health.

Raspberries are rich in vitamin C, selenium and phosphorus. Research shows they are beneficial in controlling blood sugar in diabetics. They are a great source of quercetin that is known to slow the onset and growth of cancer cells.

Blackberries are incredibly high in antioxidants and fiber and are loaded with phytochemicals that fight cancer. They are also packed with vitamin C and K.

Nuts and Seeds

Nuts and seeds are a vegan's best friend when it comes to texture, variety, healthy fats, and proteins. They are incredibly nutrient dense and contain excellent levels of fats, protein, complex carbs and fiber. They are loaded with vitamins and minerals that are easily absorbed and fun to eat, while at the same time helping to protect our bodies against disease. Every nut and seed have their own special traits:

Pine nuts have an excess amount of manganese.

Brazil nuts are the leading source of selenium

Pistachios are well known for their lutein content that supports eye health

Almonds and sunflower seeds are great sources of vitamin E.

Cashews have more iron than any other food in this category.

Pumpkin seeds are one of the best possible sources of zinc.

Olive Oil.

A staple of the Mediterranean diet for a reason, this oil is rich in antioxidants and monounsaturated fats that support cardiovascular health, prevent strokes and feed your hair and skin like nothing else. Despite being fat, it actually supports healthy weight maintenance.

Mushrooms

The best vegan meat source there is but they're low in calories while being high in protein and fiber. They're a great source of B vitamins, vitamin D, potassium and selenium. They are high in antioxidants, support healthy gut bacteria and are beneficial in weight loss.

Seaweed

Used in medicine for centuries, seaweed has antiviral properties and has recently tested positively in killing certain cancer cells. Seaweed benefits cholesterol levels and is rich in antioxidants that are proven to lower the instance of heart disease. Seaweed is incredibly rich in vitamin A, C, D, E and K, and also B vitamins. It's brimming with iron and iodine which is essential for thyroid function, as well as having decent amounts of calcium, copper, potassium, and magnesium.

Garlic

Garlic is a powerful medicinal ally to have on hand. It is rich in vitamins B6 and C, but most importantly, it boosts immune function, lowers blood pressure, improves cholesterol levels and supports cardiovascular health. Fresh garlic is brimming with antioxidants that have a potent effect on overall health.

Avocado

Avocado is a great source of MUFAs (Mono-Unsaturated Fatty Acids) which is a huge factor in cardiovascular function. They support vitamin and mineral absorption, healthy skin, hair, and eyes, improved digestive function and also contains twenty vitamins and minerals. Avocados provide anti-inflammatory activity and are loaded with soluble fiber.

Turmeric

Highly anti-inflammatory and has potent anti-cancer properties. It has been shown to provide pain relief in arthritic conditions and supports liver health due to its high antioxidant levels. Turmeric can be hard to absorb however so taking it with black pepper improves its absorptivity.

Chia Seeds

These tiny seeds are packed full of omega 3 fatty acids, in fact, they are one of the best vegan sources out there. They are also antioxidant rich and packed with protein, calcium, iron and soluble fiber. Due to this, they are recommended to reduce the occurrence of cardiovascular disease, diabetes, and obesity. They are healing to the digestive tract, contribute to feelings of fullness so support weight loss, they can help lower cholesterol and best of all, when mixed with water, they make a great egg substitute.

Legumes

A study was conducted that investigated what the longest living people and cultures in the world had in common. The only dietary thing they shared was that legumes were a huge part of their diet, in fact, the longest living people in the world at these every day. Legumes are rich in protein, fiber, and complex carbohydrates but also contain potassium, magnesium, folate, iron, B vitamins, zinc, copper, manganese, and phosphorus. These little guys are highly nutritious and loaded with soluble fiber that benefits colon health, feed healthy bacteria and reduce the risk of colon cancer.

Spirulina

Spirulina is a blue-green alga that is brimming with vitamins, minerals, and antioxidants. Algae is the greens of the sea and pack the same benefits as vegetables of the land in terms of being nutrient dense, but something about growing under the sea makes them like the Superman of vegetables. They are a great supplemental form of protein but also contain potassium, magnesium, calcium, iron, phosphorous, vitamins A and C. They benefit the cardiovascular system by lowering the risk of cholesterol and high blood pressure. They also play a role in mental health by supporting serotonin production while working simultaneously to help eliminate heavy metals and toxins from the body.

6. Foods To Avoid

There are five main food categories you will slowly want to wean out of your diet to reap the full benefits of a whole foods plant-based diet. The following categories offer little value to your health and also harm the environment.

a) Refined grains

Refined grains make up a majority of most people's diets. These tend to mainly include:

white bread

white flour

white pasta

white rice

They are referred to as 'refined' because they go through a stripping process where the fiber and most nutrients are taken out of their natural forms to increase its shelf life. This leaves you with a food product that lacks nutrients yet is loaded with calories. These types of grains have been shown to increase the risk of heart disease, diabetes, and obesity.

b) Added sugar

Sugar is frequently hidden in all types of food. Many food labels list a number of sugar sources to make it seem as though the product doesn't include as much sugar as it actually does. Since labels list ingredients from greatest to least, in quantity, you will often discover two or three sugar sources such as:

fructose

glucose

sucrose

cane sugar

beet sugar

corn syrup

sorghum syrup

Even though you may not see sugar clearly labeled as is the case with many products claiming to be healthy for you, these hidden sugars can add up when combined together. Added sugars can affect your health in a number of ways from tooth decay to an increased risk of heart disease. Since there are no health benefits to consuming added sugar, the whole foods plant-based diet excludes these items and can help you reduce your sugar cravings by supplying you with natural sugars found in many fruits. Foods you should begin to eliminate from your diet include:

sodas

fruit juices

table sugar

sugar cereals

candies

pastries

cakes

cookies

c) **Artificial sweeteners**

Artificial sweeteners are believed to be a healthier alternative to processed sugar but that is up for debate. This is why many individuals switch from regular sodas to diet sodas. Artificial sweeteners can trick the brain into thinking that the body is consuming sugar which triggers the glycemic response, in turn spiking up insulin and glucose levels. When this occurs too frequently without glucose actually being produced, which is the case when you consume artificial sweeteners, your body can develop insulin resistance which can result in developing type 2 diabetes. Aside from this major health concern, artificial sweeteners can also increase your risk of high blood pressure, obesity, heart disease, and stroke among others. A whole food plant-based diet excludes all types of artificial sweeteners such as:

splenda

sweet 'n' low

equal

nutrasweet

advantame

On food labels, these types of artificial sweeteners can be listed under the names of:

aspartame

acesulfame potassium

saccharin

sucralose

neotame

d) Packaged foods

Packaged foods are often loaded with sugars, unhealthy fats, artificial ingredients, and refined carbohydrates. These ingredients on their own have serious negative health effects and when combined can cause a great deal of damage from prolonged consumption. Many packaged foods are created to increase cravings which leads to overconsumption. In addition, most have little to no nutritional value or fiber. These products can be digested quickly in the body because of their lack of fiber content and only minimal energy is needed to process them. This is why you will often feel hungrier shortly after eating packaged foods. There is nothing about packaged foods that aligns with a whole foods plant-based diet and therefore should be avoided. Packaged foods include:
chips

frozen meals

crackers

breakfast bars

snack foods

instant meals or microwaveable meals.

e) **Processed foods**

Processed foods include a number of items where the natural nutrients that should be found have been removed. This is the case with many vegetable oils and refined flours. Even though most oils are derived from plant sources it is the Directions used to extract these oils that make them unhealthy. Extraction Directions tend to strip the nutrients from the oil so all you are left with is the fat which contains a significant amount of calories with little nutritional benefits. Plant-based oils like coconut oil, extra virgin olive oil, or sunflower oil are said to be healthier options to cook. While they may provide you with some benefits, it does not mean you need to include them in your diet every day.

Many processed foods also include chemical additives that help prolong the shelf life and improve the taste. This comes in the form of sugars, salts, and fats. Even healthy food options can be highly processed such as vegan butter, faux cheese, and tofu turkey. While you get the impression that these items may be better for you since they are labeled as vegan, they are often not good for your health.

Processed animal products are some of the most commonly consumed processed foods. These include bacon, sausages, and pre-packaged deli meats. Eating a diet that contains large amounts of processed foods puts you at risk of heart disease, diabetes, obesity, and high blood pressure.

There are a few food groups that you do not need to completely eliminate from a whole foods plant-based diet, but they should be minimally consumed. While animal meats, dairy, eggs, and seafood can have nutritional value, they can also increase the risk of disease, especially those related to blood pressure, the heart, and cholesterol levels. In the next chapter, you will learn which foods you should try your best to replace with plant-based alternatives.

7. Shopping List And Sample Menu

One important thing that will help you to start and maintain a healthy lifestyle through a plant-based diet is knowing what type of food and food ingredients should come into your plant-based diet shopping list. With this, it will be very easy for you to identify and pick varieties of whole food/plant-based food materials/ingredients which you can use while preparing your plant-based meals.

In case you usually find it very difficult to choose between what to buy and what to avoid while shopping for plant-based ingredients in the grocery stores, here is a complete shopping list for your plant-based diet. This shopping list will definitely guide you from making unhealthy choices for your plant-based meal.

1. Soy milk.

It is safer to replace the cream or milk in your coffee with soy milk, which is known to be a major carrier of protein. In a single cup of soy milk, the protein content is estimated to be about 7g, and this is enough to cater for your plant-based protein needs.

2. Almond milk

Another better alternative to dairy milk in your plant-based diet shopping list is almond milk. Almond milk is a great source of healthy fats which is a perfect and healthier substitute for dairy milk.

3. Coconut milk

A lot of people can hardly tell that coconut milk contains about 50% more calcium when compared to dairy milk. For this reason, coconut milk is a great cream as well as in smoothies. More so, you can use coconut milk to step up the tastiness of baked plant-based products.

4. Cashew milk

In case you are a strong fan of how cashews taste, you may want to add some creamy cashew milk to your shopping list. With this, you easily help yourself to avoid any appearance of dairy milk which may contradict your plant-based diet.

5. Rice milk

Another amazing plant-based product that show make it into your shopping list is rice milk. Apart from being non-allergenic, rice milk has a very low-fat content. Most importantly, rice milk has a very high vitamin b6, copper, niacin, magnesium as well as iron content.

6. Oat milk

Although a relatively new alternative to dairy milk, oat milk is very rich in protein. Oat milk contains about 4g of protein in each serving with relatively high fiber content. Oat milk is one of the healthy source of fiber and protein which is very safe for your plant-based diet shopping list.

7. Hemp milk

Hemp milk is another source of complete protein. Hemp milk is known to also contain as many omega-3 fats as your body will require for a whole day, and all these you can enjoy from just a single serving. Looking at cutting off dairy milk completely? You can replace that with hemp milk which is healthier and safer for your health.

8. Hummus

Hummus is known to be an amazing vegan dip together with some veggies or chips. Hummus can even serve as a better substitute for your mayo when preparing a crunchy veggie sandwich. Like i always tell my client, every bite of this crunchy sandwich with hummus will lead you to an irresistible indulgence in each bite (it's a permitted indulgence, though).

9. Leafy greens

You don't have to follow a plant-based diet before leafy greens make it into your shopping list. Leafy greens such as kale are must-haves for most healthy meals. Why are they so important in your meal? A cup of chopped kale is enough to provide you with high amount of vitamin a, c and k.

10.   Edamame

To most people, getting enough protein when on plant-based diet seems impossible. Well, this isn't true, and possibly because plan-based protein sources as rarely advertised. Whether you are cutting down or avoiding meat completely, a cup of edamame is enough to provide your body with a whopping 17g of protein. As a matter of fact, edamame is a super-clean snack that shouldn't be missing in your shopping list.

11.   Frozen fruit

Adding some low-budget frozen fruit into your shopping list is a big plus to your plant-based diet. One unique thing about frozen fruits is the fact that irrespective of season, anyone you lay your hands on comes pack-filled with vitamins as well as antioxidants. For instance, berries are known to be brain food which should always be a part of your smoothies.

12.   Nutritional yeast

While writing your plant-based shopping list, nutritional yeast must not be missing. Nutritional yeast serves as a better option to replace cheese, especially due to its similarity to cheese in terms of texture and flavor. Sprinkle nutritional yeast on your popcorn or your pasta to make a vegan mac n' cheese with it.

13.   Quinoa

Quinoa is a heavy weight protein carrier with lots of essential minerals and vitamins. Quinoa also serves as a delicious base when preparing some vegetable stir-fry.

14.   Bananas

Incorporating banana into your shopping list can serve as a better alternative for one egg in pancakes and cakes.

15.   Blackstrap molasses

If you are in need of a source of dairy-free calcium, blackstrap molasses can be the best ingredient to include in your shopping list.

16.   Cashews

Just like nutritional yeast, you can use cashews as cheesy topping for all your vegan meals. Alternatively, you can make cashew cream to go with every bowl of pasta. Better still, you may decide to make a raw carrot cake using cashew cream cheese. The varieties you can get from cashew is almost unending

17.   Almonds

Your plant-based diet may not be complete with almonds. It will interest you to know that almonds are great sources of manganese as well as vitamin e. Just with a hand, almonds can become an enjoyable and healthy snack.

18.   Organic sprouted grain bread

Sure, you didn't know that most bread contains milk ingredients. So, this is the reason why your plant-based shopping list should contain only organic sprouted grain bread. Doing this won't only save your plant-based diets lifestyle, it will also help you to avoid the chances of eating a dairy product.

19.   Seaweed

For all vegans, sea weed is a must! Seaweed are rich in omega-3-fatty acids, and so, you can use that as a good excuse to opt for more sensational seaweed salad during a sushi night outing.

20.   Dry lentils

With lentils, you are sure of about 18g of protein and 16g of fiber in a single cup. Using some dry lentils with quinoa for your burger can be a better and healthier alternative when you are craving for some juicy burger.

21.   Carrots

Without much hassles, you can enjoy carrots in a wide variety such as steamed, raw, roasted or even in baked goods. One good reason why carrots shouldn't be missing in you plant-based diet shopping list is because carrots are rich in vitamin a, c, beta-carotene as well a heavy-weight fiber carrier.

22.   Beets

Beets contains a lot of flavor with radiant colours that can lighten up your dish and it can even serve as a healthy and tasty appetizer.

23.   Artichokes

Another spicy ingredient to add into your plant-based diet shopping list is artichokes. Artichokes are known to have a strong zesty flavor, and they are great and healthy addition into your bowl of veggies. Nutritionally, artichokes are rich sources of protein which just half a cup can offer up to about 4g of proteins.

24.   Asparagus

There are tons of plant-based sources of protein, and one of them which you can pick from the grocery store is asparagus. With a deep hue of green colouration, asparagus are rich in flavor with packs of protein as well as vitamins b6, folate and potassium.

25.   Tempeh

Tempeh is yet another fermented soybean product with a tough texture and nutty taste which makes it a perfect option when you need some plant-based source of protein. For instance, maple glazed temper with kale and quinoa is an amazing, clean and delicious source of vegan protein.

26.   Coconut oil

It is no secret that the most-revered coconut oil is a better option to use for your baking or cooking instead of butter. So, when you have the urge to scoop some butter into your fries, coconut oil will do the job perfectly, instead.

27.   Avocado

Avocados are silent plant-based diet ingredient with lots of health benefits. So, when next you need something with a creamy texture and your thought reminds you of some dairy products, simply grad a ball of avocado, and you are better off with that. Interestingly, avocados are packed with healthy fats, vitamin b6, fiber, protein, potassium as well as magnesium.

28.   Cauliflower

One of the most versatile cruciferous vegetable known to me is cauliflower. It can go well with pizza crust, mashed potatoes, or even as the major ingredient in when preparing a coconut curry dish.

29.   Squash

If you need to boost your omega-3-fatty acids, squash is one fruit that you can enjoy in so many forms in your diet. With a characteristic taste like a vegetable, squash contains a high amount of vitamin b, potassium and iron. For people who are staunch soup lovers, a slow cooker carrot squash soup can sure make their day.

30.   Mushrooms

When you need a better alternative to meat in your plant-based diet, mushrooms can make a perfect choice. With their meaty texture as well as a high level of juiciness, you can tell that mushroom is enough to satisfy your cravings for a bite of beef.

31.   Oats

When you need some healthy dose of plant-based protein to get you energized and satisfied all day, oats can be that perfect item that you must include in your shopping list.

32.   Amaranth

Although a less popular grain, amaranth is a sweet and nutty grain with amazing flavor. A cup of amaranth is enough to fill you with about 6g of protein. Amaranth is one of the clean and healthy breakfast cereals you should have in your shopping list.

33.   Buckwheat

For people with gluten intolerance, buckwheat flour is another good alternative to harness all the protein and magnesium that your body needs for energy and vitality.

34.   Teff

Only if you can look beyond the size, teff pack punch of protein in its tiny seeds. Teff is also another alternative for a gluten-free cooking.

35.   Flax, chia, and hemp seeds

Here are seeds that are packed with iron, magnesium, fiber and omega-3-fats. Adding flax, chia or hemps seeds into your morning salad, baked into cookies or even in your smoothie is a good and healthy way to start a great day.

36.   Sunflower seeds

Sunflower seeds are rich in vitamin e which is known to enhance focus and energy. So, you can add them into your snacks when you need to boost your energy level.

37.   Walnuts

Another plant-based ingredient that your shopping list should have is walnuts. Either ground or in their raw form, walnuts are a great source of magnesium, vitamin e and omega-3- fats.

38.   Aquafaba

I am sure that you may be sceptic about aquafaba as it may sound very strange to you. Well, it may be a familiar dietary ingredient, but i bet that you'll be glad to hear about its enormous health benefits here. Aquafaba is another good plant-based ingredient that you should include into your shopping list.

Aquafaba is the high-starch liquid which is present in a can of cooked chickpeas. Aquafaba is also known to be a great foaming and thickening agent. If you've been on the lookout for a safer alternative to eggs, i am confident to let you know that aquafaba is a better substitute. With a tablespoon of aquafaba, you can confidently assure yourself of having taken one egg yolk and two tablespoons of aquafaba is equivalent to one egg white.

39.　　　　　　　Seitan

Have you been looking for a way to cut off all forms of gluten in your plant-based diet? Then adding seitan to your shopping list can turn out to be the best and safest escape route from gluten. Seitan has a chewy texture, and it blends perfectly with a lot of spices. Nutritionally, seitan is rich in protein and free from cholesterol.

40.　　　　　　　Sweet potato

Sweet potato is one plant-based product which shouldn't be found missing in your shopping list. Sweet potato is a very nutritious food which is packed with lots of cancer-fighting beta carotene. If you need to give yourself an out of the box experience, you may want to try roasted sweet potatoes with turmeric and cardamom recipe in your plant-based diet.

41.   Veggie sausages

Have been eating faux meats? If yes, then you need to know that faux meats are loaded with lots of processed ingredients. You can safe your body such with a healthier alternative such as field roast brand. Also, you can substitute turkey sausage with some veggies sausage like fennel and sausage stuffing filled with pepper which is a better alternative as a good plant-based meal.

42.   Veggie burgers

Veggie burgers such as black bean superfood burgers are pretty simple to prepare. Besides being easy to make, they are also delicious and healthy for your plant-based diet.

43.   Soy yogurt

Including some soy yoghurt in your plant-based shopping list is one way to show your gut more love. In case you never knew, soy yoghurt is filled with probiotics which are healthy microbes that enhances the health of your gut.

44.   Agar agar

Agar agar is another great substitute for gelatin if you hope to be a staunch and faithful vegan. It is a healthy ingredient you should add to your plant-based diet shopping list.

45.   Miso paste

If you ever thought of plant-based food as being bland, then you are wrong. With miso paste, you can step up your plant-based shopping list, as it serves as a better substitute for anchovy and also adds umami to vegetables.

46.   Vegetable broth

Instead of using just water, you can include vegetable broth in your shopping list. Vegetable broth happens to be a perfect replacement for water as it adds some enticing flavor to your meal, especially when cooking quinoa.

47.   Tomato paste

As common as tomato paste may be, it is a good source of iron besides being that ingredient that adds a red hue to your lentil stew. Tomato paste is also a good ingredient for your plant-based diet shopping list as it also contributes to stepping up the flavor of your meal.

48.   Sun-dried tomatoes

Looking for a way to increase texture and flavor? Sun-dried tomatoes is another spicy ingredient to have around in your kitchen. So, make sure it isn't missing in your plant-based shopping list.

49.   Capers

Another flavored and salty addition to your plant-based meals is capers.

50.   Tahini or sesame paste

Sesame paste or tahini is yet another great plant-based condiment which is very rich in dietary minerals such as lecithin, potassium, phosphorus, iron and magnesium.

8. What Is Wrong With Eating Processed Foods?

A better question would be, "what isn't wrong with eating processed foods?" Simply put, processed foods are bad for you. They are a no-no. And that fact cannot be overstated. Here's the thing; processed foods have been altered to improve their appearance, improve their taste and extend their shelf life. In order to accomplish this, manufacturers add a bunch of chemicals (over 6,000 unnatural chemicals are found in processed foods) to color, flavor, sweeten, stabilize, texturize, bleach, emulsify, preserve, soften and hide odors.

In other words, by the time they're done, the processed foods have been stripped down of their nutrients and turned into something that should frankly not be allowed in the markets. Most general grocery stores are filled with isles and isles of processed foods and rarely anything we should actually be putting in our bodies. I find when I go to a general store like "Ralphs" or "Safeway" I shop the produce section, a few items here and there and find the **Ezekiel sprouted bread**. I am a huge advocate of farmer's markets instead.

But that's not all.

Processed foods found in the grocery store have been linked to a variety of health issues. These include:

1: Obesity. With over one third of the world's population estimated to be obese or overweight, it is evident that obesity is a problem. What you may not know is that processed food is its cheerleader! How is that so? Well, for starters, processed food is made to be *hyper rewarding* thanks to its high concentration of simple carbohydrates that excite the reward centers of the brain. In fact, when you eat processed foods, your brain 'rejoices', your dopamine receptors are flooded and you end up craving this taste and rush again. The body and brain feels the urge to get a new dose of this glucose boost to feel that surge of "happy". This is why many people are addicted to sweet, fatty and salty processed foods. The taste buds and brain receptors go crazy for it. To your brain, it's like taking a feel-good drug. That's not all; processed foods are tasty and manufacturers outdo each other to keep them that way. As a result, once you consume them, you find yourself eating more and more. For some reason, you can't stop eating until there's no more food left. All these factors i.e. the fact that they are high in carbohydrates and trigger strong cravings greatly push us to a point of overindulgence, which in turn triggers weight gain. Not to mention, your body has a hard time breaking these processed foods down. These carbohydrates make us fat and the excess carbs are converted into fatty acids and glycerol then stored in different fat stores around the body if we do not burn them off consistently.

2: Diabetes. There is a very good reason why people with Type II Diabetes are advised to change their diet in order to reverse the disease. What you eat matters. More precisely, diabetics are told to avoid foods high in sugars (carbohydrates) to ensure they don't increase their blood sugar to dangerous levels. I've seen diabetes kill people close to me, and I've seen my friends young and old become diagnosed with diabetes. I don't want you to get to the point of being told by doctors you have to minimize or avoid foods that are high in sugars and carbohydrates like processed foods, in fear of being taken by this reversible and life-style based disease. A scary fact is that by 2050 1/3rd of our population will have diabetes. Please don't let it be you.

If you are a fan of processed foods, you increase your risk of getting Type 2 Diabetes. For one, the more you consume such foods, the more you elevate your blood sugar levels since these tend to be high in carbohydrates. What you may not know is that having high blood sugar levels over an extended period can make your cells less receptive to insulin. And insulin is a hormone produced by the beta cells of the pancreas in response to rising blood glucose. The higher the blood glucose (as a result of eating foods high in carbohydrates), the more insulin needs to be produced. The body cells have no internal mechanism of taking up glucose/sugar from the bloodstream. They need help and this help is offered by insulin. The purpose of insulin therefore is to act as some sort of key that triggers the cells to open up so as to take up blood glucose for use in energy. This process is very efficient since it helps the cells to remove glucose from the bloodstream before the next meal. Unfortunately, if you have high blood glucose concentrations all the time, the cells keep being bombarded by insulin. Keep in mind that the higher the glucose, the higher the insulin. This is not good because it can easily make the cells go 'deaf' (or simply less sensitive) to insulin, which we need to live and regulate our food to energy conversion. Think of this as hearing the same high pitched sound all the time; you will soon not respond with the same urgency. The same thing happens to the cells. When this happens, the body responds by upping the amount of insulin that it produces to make the cells hear the message. In other words, the insulin has to be a bit 'louder' for the cells to get the message. This is what's referred to as insulin resistance and is the precursor to diabetes. Over an extended period, this excessive production can push the body to a point where it impairs the beta cells of the pancreas. Ultimately, you may end up having a hard time managing blood glucose and this is what is referred to as Diabetes.

3: Heart disease. Another good reason to shun processed foods is that they tend to be high in trans-fat and unhealthy, processed vegetable oils. Such fats contain an excess of omega-6 fatty acids. Taking too much of these could increase your likelihood of developing such health problems as inflammation, oxidation and an increased risk of heart disease.

Unfortunately, given that trans fats and seed oils are very common, this perhaps explains why heart disease is ranked at the top when it comes to cause of death in Western countries.

Thus, if you want to successfully adopt the plant based diet, please stay away from processed oils, wheat, flour, meat and dairy. These products created in factories and labs only end up killing us. The convenience you may get from using such foods is definitely not worth it in the long run. I know it can be difficult at first, and at first we will definitely still crave things like cheese and bread. For cheese I recommend finding vegan substitutes like cashew cheese. They can also be made of sesame seeds, **coconut oil**, almonds and nutritional yeast. It may take a little more searching but you can find them in the vegan isle, health food stores and even **plant based parmesan on Amazon**! And if you still want to enjoy eating breads and sandwiches, go for **sprouted** bread!

9. Planning Plant-Based Meals

Has it ever happened to you to go home after a busy day, to inspect your refrigerator with a blank stare, and ask, "what are we going to eat tonight?". It is at this time of the day that many people decide to get food delivered or opt for a really easy solution for dinner, such as making a sandwich. Once again. But there is a way to make sure you have something good to eat at the end of a long day. The secret is to plan with plant-based meals.

Meal planning allows you to know in advance which meals will be served on weekday evenings. This helps prepare a shopping list, minimizing ready-to-eat meals and putting vegetables on the menu. Planning well also allows you to get ahead and prepare some dishes before you even start the week. But above all, it helps to clear the head of the famous question: "what are we eating tonight?

Planning your plant-based meals helps you to eat well, to have a meal delivered less often (and thus to save you money!), and, in addition, it helps you to be less stressed about what you are going to eat.

Here are some things you can do to enjoy delicious, well-prepared plant-based meals:

Why plan your plant-based meals?

Planning your plant-based meals has many benefits and allows you to:

To avoid decisional fatigue

When it's time for dinner, you've spent the day making decisions big or small. Having to decide what you are going to eat at the last minute is additional stress that may lead you to draw pasta (or pizza delivery) for the umpteenth time!

By deciding in a quiet moment - the weekend for example - of your plant-based meals of the week, you will not have the evening only but also launch in the realization. It's simply liberating!

To limit food waste

Planning plant-based meals are also taking the time to take stock of what you already have in your refrigerator, your freezer, your cupboard (or even your garden) and must be consumed more or less quickly. By the way, you will save money.

To eat more varied and balanced

By having visibility of several days on your meals, you will be able to identify the foods that come back often and that you could perhaps replace.

To get ahead

To have in mind or under the eyes the menus of the days to come also encourages to do small tasks ahead of time, such as to clean a salad or plants, to put tofu to marinate. Little things in the evening will have saved you precious time.

How to plan your meals?

I do not believe that there is an infallible and universal Directions. The right Directions is the one that suits you: you do not find it compelling, and it makes your life easier. The key is to get started without waiting to find the Directions. A sheet of paper and a pencil are enough!

Start by taking a calendar

Write down your professional and social commitments, school events, and anything that affects your schedule. If you share your meals with family members or friends, also consider their schedule on the calendar. Then see the days when you'll have time to cook, and the days you'll have less time. Opt for meals that will go with the time you have. For example, if you see that you will only have 10 minutes on a certain day, you can expect to cook something in that regard, not a chicken and roast potatoes.

Choose recipes and go grocery shopping

Find plant-based meal ideas for each night, and list the ingredients you will need. Go grocery shopping with your list in hand to stock up. Having basic foods will make it easy for you, and you'll be able to prepare the week's dinners quickly. This will also save you time because you will not have to run to the grocery store every day. And because you'll know what to cook every night, you can open your fridge and start cooking once you're home.

Cook new recipes

Interest in books, magazines and cooking shows continues to grow, and many parents have multiple home cooking books at home. But how often are these new recipes on the menu?

When planning the menu of the week, this is the perfect time to flip through your books and put inspiring recipes on the menu. At the same time, you make the shopping list. Make sure to read the recipe, if it requires marinating the meat 12 hours in advance, it will be necessary to foresee it.

If you cook especially at the last minute, it is often the same recipes that will be on the menu because they are the ones you know to do by heart. If they come back too often, you will always feel like eating the same thing. By including new recipes, the menu will be more varied, and it will also be more motivating to cook.

By planning meals well, it will also be possible to try to incorporate new dishes and foods on the menu — for example, vegetarian meals or a new vegetable.

Classic planning

You choose recipes and place them in your plan, then you draw up a shopping list based on that. This Directions can be optimized by using applications that offer integrated shopping lists, and you can also subscribe to meal planners who cook menus based on your preferences.

For those who want to progress and repeatedly train on a type of dish this allows you to search for ideas in a specific context, in short, you no longer go to the assault of bottomless pit recipes on the internet or even in your cookbooks without knowing where you go.

Meal planning is a key element in good food management. If you have tried several times to better plan meals, but the habit is still not anchored, there is surely something else that does not work.

Hence, the idea is to use a little of each approach while adapting to its concrete context: skills, constraints of the week, etc. Reviewing these different Directions nevertheless seemed interesting to situate your practice, and i hope you open new horizons!

10. Essential Nutrients to Consider

An important aspect of any diet plan is knowing the nutrients that you will be getting from the foods you eat. This guarantees that you don't deny your body essential nutrients it needs for growth and other purposes. Vegetarians should be mindful of the nutrients in their foods simply because of deficiency issues. In this case, you should be aware of the best foods to provide you with protein alternatives and other vital nutrients such as iron, vitamin B-12, calcium, vitamin C, zinc, and omega-3 fatty acids.

Often, most people have the perception that plant foods lack the good quality of protein that the body needs. Equally, some dieters are worried that, by sticking to a plant-based diet, they might be denying their bodies vital nutrients. It is for this very reason that this chapter will help you understand the right foods you should choose when in search of particular nutrients.

Protein

Protein is an essential nutrient in the body. It not only helps in building and repairing muscles, but it also aids in maintaining our skin and bone health. The immune system also requires protein to function optimally in warding off diseases. So, if you are new to a vegan diet, you may have questions concerning your protein sources. Of course, this is attributed to the myth that plant-based diets don't provide the body with sufficient nutrients.

However, there are several plant foods that will provide you with the protein you need in your diet. Some of these foods include beans, soy products, seeds, nuts, peas, vegetables, and whole grains. When looking for proteins in vegetables, your shopping cart should be filled with veggies like broccoli, yellow sweet corn, potatoes, lentils, green peas, Brussels sprouts, broccoli rabe, avocado, and cauliflower.

Evidently, you can see that you have plenty of options to choose from when in search of protein in your diet. Now, let's do some math to determine the amount of protein you might need in your diet. According to the Dietary Reference Intakes, the amount of protein you should consume daily is equivalent to 0.8 grams per kilogram of your body weight, or 0.36 grams per pound. Say you weigh 80 kilograms. You should multiply this by 0.8 grams to determine the protein quantity you require daily. In this case, the quantity of protein will be 64 grams.

The various foods mentioned above offer varying amounts of protein. This implies that combining several veggies together will provide you with what you need. A one cup serving of lentils, for instance, will provide you with 18 grams of protein. A cup of green peas, on the other hand, will only provide you with 8.5 grams of protein (Chertoff, 2016). Judging from the numbers, all you need is a mix of different plant foods to meet your daily protein intake.

Iron

There are various functions of iron in our bodies. This makes this nutrient very important. The nutrient is required for blood production. It also aids in the transportation of oxygen in the blood through the production of hemoglobin. Lack of iron in the blood will result in the body not obtaining sufficient oxygen. The presence of iron in the body also guarantees that the food we eat is easily converted into energy (Spatone, "What Does Iron Do for the Body? The Role of Iron: Spatone"). It is also worth mentioning that the body requires iron for optimal cognitive function. Brain functions that depend on iron include alertness, attention, memory, intelligence, problem-solving, and learning. Therefore, a balanced intake of iron ensures that our brains function well.

The above-mentioned benefits of iron prove that iron is indeed an important nutrient that the body requires. Unfortunately, the body doesn't naturally produce iron. Consequently, it is up to us to supplement it through good food choices. Plant foods that provide us with iron include legumes, nuts and seeds, grains, and vegetables.

Ideal legumes to shop for are lentils, tofu, lima beans, chickpeas, black beans, and soybeans. The best grains to shop for here include fortified cereals, oatmeal, brown rice, and quinoa. In terms of nuts and seeds, you should go for pine, squash, pumpkin, sunflower, cashews, and pistachios. Collard greens, Swiss chard, and tomato sauce are also excellent sources of iron in the vegetable category.

Vitamin B12

Like iron, vitamin B12 is an essential nutrient required for optimal functioning of the brain. Additionally, it helps in the production of red blood cells. This vitamin is not present in plant foods. However, it can easily be obtained in meat. Since you are switching sides, it is imperative to know where you can get this nutrient.

The absence of vitamin B12 in plant foods shouldn't discourage you from strictly avoiding animal-based products. As a vegan, you should consider taking supplements to provide you with this nutrient. If you are going to do this, ensure that you discuss this with your physician and them recommend the best supplements.

However, the vitamin can be found in fortified foods including cereals, nutritional yeast, hemp milk, and meat substitutes. Before purchasing these products from the stores, it is vital that you read the nutrition labels. This way, you avoid taking home foods high in sugar and other unhealthy oils.

Calcium

When you think of calcium, the first thing that comes to mind is milk, right? Well, over the years, we have been made to understand that dairy foods are the best sources of calcium. While this is true, you should also realize that the nutrient can be obtained from plant foods. To avoid the negative health effects associated with dairy and other animal products, it is best to choose certain plant foods.

Calcium is of great importance to our bone health and teeth development. It also has a role to play in nerve signaling, muscle function, and heart health. Adults should ingest 1,000 mg of calcium daily. Children should have an even higher intake of 1,300 mg daily (Jennings, 2018).

Ideal plant-based sources of calcium include bok choy, Chinese cabbage, broccoli, calcium-set tofu, beans, lentils, and fruits. The best fruits here include blackberries, blackcurrants, and raspberries.

Vitamin C

Vitamin C will be an easier nutrient to obtain since most fruits and vegetables can provide the body with this vital nutrient. This vitamin helps in strengthening the body's immune system. As a result, vitamin C is often perceived as a remedy for the common cold. Recommended vegan foods to add to your diet here include broccoli, pineapple, Brussels sprouts, kiwi, bell peppers, oranges, and spinach. All of these foods provide you with varying quantities of vitamin C. For instance, a one cup serving of broccoli will provide you with about 81 mg of vitamin C. A higher quantity can be gained from a cup of kiwi since it provides you with nearly 167 mg of the nutrient (Von Alt, 2017).

Zinc

Zinc has several important functions in the body. It is ranked as an essential nutrient because the body cannot naturally produce it. Hence, it is worth knowing how you can supplement your diet to ensure that you provide your body with this nutrient. Zinc comes second as the most abundant mineral in the body after iron (Kubala, 2018). The mineral helps with metabolism, nerve function, digestion, and immune functions.

So, which foods should you eat to get zinc? Ideal sources include tempeh, whole grains, tofu, lentils, seeds, nuts, peas, beans, and several fortified cereals. In some cases, zinc might not be easily absorbed by the body due to phytates compounds. Therefore, it is highly recommended that you soak some of these foods before cooking. Grains, seeds, and beans fall in this category.

Omega-3 Fatty Acids

Omega-3 fatty acids are also essential nutrients, meaning that the body cannot produce them. There are three forms of omega-3 fatty acids:

- Docosahexaenoic acid (DHA)

- Alpha-linolenic acid (ALA)

- Eicosapentaenoic acid (EPA)

Individuals who eat fish usually obtain DHA and EPA. ALA, on the other hand, is obtained from plant foods. The good news is that the body can convert ALA obtained from plants into DHA and EPA. However, the process is not as efficient. Consequently, you could supplement your diet with hemp seed oil, flaxseed oil, or chia seeds to aid in optimizing the conversion process.

Other recommended foods to ingest include algal oil, walnuts, perilla oil, and Brussels sprouts.

The information detailed in this section should help you realize that important nutrients that are often assumed to be present only in animal products can also be obtained from plant foods. Therefore, knowing and understanding the nutrients you are getting from your plant foods is important; it confirms that you are getting all the vital nutrients your body requires for optimal functioning.

11. Fully Transition

Getting rid of meat is the first step in fully transitioning to a plant-based diet. But there are other things you still need to do. Remember, your goal is to fully transition to a plant-based diet as soon as you can. This will give your body enough time to adjust to the diet and you'll be able to see the benefits of sticking to the diet. As such, you need to:

Get rid of eggs and dairy

A lot of people think that giving up dairy is the one thing that can stop them from embracing a plant-based diet. But it can be done. Think about it. Less than 40% of adults have the ability to digest lactose. If you can't digest lactose, you'll be faced with issues such as flatulence, bloating, diarrhea, cramping and nausea. This is because the sugars you consume will get stuck in the colon and they will begin to ferment. As such, you have added reason to stop consuming dairy.

Another thing you need to stop eating is eggs. Yes, this includes the eggs you use in baking. Instead of using eggs, you can use things such as flax eggs, banana and chia eggs.

Rethink how you shop

Now that you've gotten rid of meat, eggs and dairy, it is time to rethink how you shop. Start by clearing out your pantry. Get rid of any food product that should not be consumed in the plant-based diet. Next, think of what you need to purchase and where you're likely to get it. Instead of browsing the supermarket isles, you may need to change tactics and head to the farmers markets and farms whenever possible. This way, you'll get fresh produce at lower prices. Don't waste time on things you can no longer eat. Avoid such sections if you can. A list of what you need will come in handy.

You also need to familiarize yourself with the practice of checking labels. Remember, you are now on the plant-based diet. Animal products should not have a place in your shopping list. Reading labels will help you see any red flags and as such, you'll be able to avoid such products.

Stock your pantry

You should make it a habit to stock your pantry with the types of food you want to eat. As they say, out of sight, out of mind. If you want to add certain foods in your diet, you need to be able to reach for them whenever you need them. Foods such as fruits, vegetables, whole grains, healthy fats, legumes, nuts and seeds should all have a place in your pantry. It would certainly help to have a few recipes nearby so that you can plan for what you'll need to buy.

Don't go overboard when you are shopping. You don't need to stock your pantry with foods you won't eat. It would be wiser to find a few foods you intend to use frequently and make sure you have enough of them. For example, you can shop in bulk for things such as rice and oats and decide to shop weekly for things such as fresh fruits and vegetables. As time goes by, you'll have a good idea of how much food you'll be eating and your shopping will become easier.

What to expect: after 20 days

In the first two weeks, you should have fully transitioned to the plant-based diet. After 20 days, you can check your progress to see if you are on the right track. There are certain things you'll notice after 20 days on the plant-based diet.

Once you fully switch to the plant-based diet, you should expect to have bad days. Yes, there are days that will be more difficult than others. This is especially so in the first few days of fully transitioning. You'll crave certain foods. You'll crave animal products and start 'dreaming about' foods you can no longer eat. This is normal. But as days go by, the cravings will subside. Something else that you'll notice is that your taste buds will 'come alive'. The various foods you'll be eating will contribute to a boost in taste and sensation. You need to give yourself time to adjust before determining whether or not you like a certain type of food.

On a positive note, you'll soon notice that you have a lot of energy. This energy will be consistent throughout the day. It won't fluctuate. Things like afternoon 'slumps' will be things of the past. If you were used to sleeping in the course of the day, you'll find that you are more alert throughout the day. As such, your days will become more productive. If you take advantage of this, you'll be able to experience improved sleep during the night.

Once you give up eggs and dairy, you'll notice a change in how you feel. If your body was constantly experiencing aches and pains, you'll find relief. This is because the foods you'll be eating will be full of anti-inflammatory properties. They will help you get rid of chronic pain.

As you fully embrace the diet, you may find yourself fielding questions from your friends and family. People will be curious and some will be suspicious as they see the changes you are making. They will have questions and some may discourage you and make fun of you. This should not stop you from completing the program. This is the time to remind yourself of your motivations and while you're on it, you need to learn to upgrade the diet.